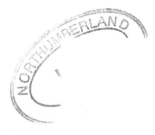
INTRODUCTION TO
Paddling

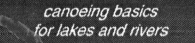

*canoeing basics
for lakes and rivers*

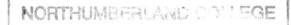

Acknowledgments

Earlier versions of this booklet were published as *Flat-Water Paddler* by the Ohio Department of Natural Resources' Division of Watercraft. The American Canoe Association thanks the Ohio DNR for its generosity in granting use of the earlier work, and for its cooperation in this update and revision. The ACA also thanks the United States Coast Guard for support in the development and implementation of the *Introduction to Paddling* and *Introduction to River Paddling* curricula through an Aquatics Resources Trust Fund (Wallop-Breaux) grant. These curricula served as the basis for deciding what to include and exclude in this revision.

We also thank the members of the American Canoe Association revision team: Kim Whitley, National Instruction Committee Chair; Charlie Wilson, NIC Vice-Chair; Pamela Dillon, NIC secretary and Ohio DNR Watercraft Education Administrator; Virgil Chambers; and Deborah Macmillan, ACA's Director of Safety Education and Instruction.

Design by Kandace Hawkinson
Illustrations by Les Fry. Illustrations on pages 23, 24, and 25 are from previous American Canoe Association publications and are by Carol A. Moore.

ISBN 0-89732-202-9
Library of Congress Catalog Card Number applied for.

Note: Outdoor activities are an assumed risk sport. This book cannot take the place of appropriate instruction for paddling, swimming, or lifesaving techniques. Every effort has been made to make this guide as accurate as possible, but it is the ultimate responsibility of the paddler to judge his or her ability and act accordingly.

Menasha Ridge Press
3169 Cahaba Heights Road
Birmingham, AL 35243
(800) 247-9437

American Canoe Association
7432 Alban Station Blvd., Suite B-226
Springfield, VA 22150
(703) 451-0141

Table of Contents

Foreword

People take to paddling for reasons as varied as the people themselves. The canoe, rich in history and tradition, appeals to individuals, to families, and to groups. People may paddle for a quiet afternoon on a park pond or for days on end down a wilderness river. This variety helps make canoeing one of America's most popular outdoor activities.

Safe, enjoyable paddling requires both knowledge and skill. This manual will help you gain both. If canoeing skills are developed with safety in mind, paddlers can have fun and be confident. If it's not safe and fun, it's better left undone!

In addition to reading this booklet and practicing what you learn from it, we strongly recommend formal instruction. The American Canoe Association's *Introduction to Paddling* and *Introduction to River Paddling* courses emphasize safety, enjoyment, and the development of introductory paddling skills as summarized below:

AMERICAN CANOE ASSOCIATION
Introduction to Paddling and *Introduction to River Paddling*
Course Goals

SAFETY: To safely paddle on flat and moving water, perform self rescue, and respond to emergencies that arise.
ENJOYMENT: To become aware of paddling opportunities and the rewards of lifetime participation in paddling.
SKILLS: To acquire the ability to safely and enjoyably paddle on quiet and moving water.

For more information, contact:
American Canoe Association
7432 Alban Station Blvd., Suite B-226
Springfield, Va 22150
Phone: (703) 451-0141
Internet: http://www.aca-paddler.org

How to Be Safe on the Water

Canoeing is fun, but it can be risky! Let's imagine some conditions paddlers might encounter. Read the following description and then list the risks these paddlers are taking.

Early in March, Cliff arrives at Susie's house in northern Ohio with a new canoe. Susie is excited. She's never been in a canoe, and asks to go paddling that afternoon. The sun is shining with a forecast in the mid-sixties, so, dressed in cotton T-shirts and jeans, they drive to the river. The water looks high and is moving fast. It takes a long time to untie the canoe from the car, but they eventually throw paddles, life jackets and a six pack of beer into the canoe and push off. Water splashes into their canoe as they head downstream.

The description above was compiled from actual accident reports.

List the risk factors Cliff and Susie are taking. There are at least 10. (Check your answers on page 8.)

1.

2.

3.

4.

5.

6.

Now list ways to minimize these risks.

1.

2.

3.

4.

5.

6.

Become a safe paddler by reducing potential risk. Weather, water conditions, wind, temperature, equipment, prior planning, group composition, and experience all play a part in the safe boating formula. Understanding the following key points will reduce your chances of a mishap and increase your enjoyment.

LIFE JACKETS

Life jackets are also called Personal Flotation Devices, or PFDs. The American Canoe Association requires that life jackets be worn during its canoeing programs. Many states have similar requirements. Remember, most paddlers who drown were not wearing their life jackets. Life jackets provide buoyancy in the water and work best when fitted securely. Be smart. Wear your life jacket.

Contact your state boating agency to learn the laws that apply regarding life jackets and other safety equipment to be carried on board a canoe.

HYPOTHERMIA

Cold water can disable even the strongest of swimmers! Exposure to cold water can cause hypothermia, a condition which results in a lowering of your body's core temperature. It develops when the body cannot produce enough heat to keep its temperature normal. As the body's temperature drops, visible signs appear: unclear thinking, uncontrollable shivering, followed by difficulty speaking, muscular rigidity, loss of coordination, and eventually loss of consciousness, then death.

Prevention is the key. The best way to prevent hypothermia is to BE AWARE and BE PREPARED!! Wear proper clothing and a life jacket that fits! Clothing can include: a wetsuit, wool or synthetic layers, and a wool or synthetic hat. Cotton is a poor insulator when wet. When water temperature is 55 degrees Fahrenheit or below, or water and air temperatures don't add up to 100 degrees Fahrenheit, wear a wet or dry suit. Look for weather changes constantly. Be prepared and act quickly.

WIND AND WAVES

Wind produces waves on lakes. Waves can be great fun, but can lead to swamping or a capsize. Stay in protected waters unless you and your group can handle rough water and are prepared to rescue overturned boats. Wind may make it difficult for you to travel to your intended destination by either blowing you off course or slowing your progress.

RIVER READING

Moving water has awesome power. Smart paddlers understand and respect its strength. High and fast water levels caused by rain, snowmelt and dam releases are no place to learn canoeing. Fast, powerful water can push you into hazardous situations such as downed trees or other obstructions. Learn the dynamics of the river. Experienced river paddlers know how to "read the river." River reading is the ability to analyze the surface current. It helps you determine where to go and what to avoid. River reading opens the door to the fun of "river running" and playing in rapids.

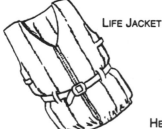
LIFE JACKET

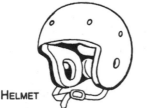
HELMET

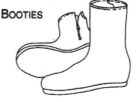
BOOTIES

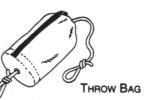
THROW BAG

Dress for the water temperature, not mid-afternoon air temperature. A layering system of clothing is important, as air trapped between layers is good insulation; adding or removing a layer of clothing allows easy comfort adjustment. Cotton clothing is questionable except in extreme heat, as cotton holds moisture when wet and cools the body. Wool and synthetic pile are much better insulators wet or dry, but need a wind and waterproof outer layer to increase their effectiveness. Proper insulation on head, hands, and feet will increase paddler comfort in cold conditions. Extreme cold requires wet suits or synthetic insulation under dry suits. Life jackets are a valuable outside insulating layer in addition to supplying flotation when in the water.

FOOTWEAR

Footwear is a critical item of paddling gear. This is not the time to go barefoot! Cuts to the feet and sprained ankles are the most common injuries among inexperienced paddlers. Whether carrying a canoe over rugged, wet and slippery terrain, or launching in ankle deep water, foot support and protection is important. Neoprene booties and old athletic shoes with wool or synthetic socks are wise choices in cold water.

KNEE PROTECTION

Kneeling in a canoe increases stability and leverage and decreases the chance of a capsize. Knee protection increases comfort. Kneepads may be worn over the knees, glued into the canoe or larger pads dropped into the canoe bottom. They should be made of closed cell, non-absorbing foam and textured for a non-slip surface.

END LINES

End lines, also called "painters," are short ropes tied to canoe ends. They can be used to tie the canoe to shore, stabilize it when on a cartop carrier, and tow it during rescues. Ideally, they should be polypropylene, 3/8" minimum diameter and about 15 feet long. Polypropylene is the best choice because it floats. While paddling, stow end lines where they are accessible but cannot loosen and entangle swimming paddlers should you capsize.

ADDITIONAL GEAR

What you carry is based on your trip's length, access to services, and group make-up. Consider taking the following: water bottle, sunglasses, sunscreen, insect repellent, first aid kit, toilet paper, compass and maps, sponge, bailer, whistle, flashlight, rescue rope and sling, knife, dry bags, extra paddle, matches, extra flotation for the canoe, duct tape, food, guide books, garbage bags, glass straps, camera, fishing gear, and emergency signaling devices.

SYNTHETIC TOP

PADDLING JACKET

PADDLING PANTS

1. What is a good rule of thumb for determining when a wet/dry suit is needed?

2. Describe criteria for dressing for a canoe trip.

3. List items appropriate to take on a canoe trip.

4. What is hypothermia? What are its early symptoms?

5. What is the leading factor in canoe drownings?

6. What are the most common canoe injuries?

Answers to Cliff and Susie's paddling risks: 1. Not wearing their life jackets; 2. Inexperience; 3. Cotton clothing won't keep them warm if they get wet; 4. Cold air/water; 5. High water; 6. Fast water; 7. Use of alcohol; 8. Not knowing river; 9. Boating alone; 10. Not informing others where they are going and when to expect their return.

Answers to minimizing Cliff and Susie's risk factors (the numbers here correspond to the numbered risk factors above): 1. Wear life jackets; 2. Take a canoeing course; 3, 4. Wear clothing for conditions; 5, 6. Read a river guide book and observe the skills needed for the existing water level; 7. Avoid the use of alcohol; 8, 9. Boat with others who know the river and are more experienced; 10. File a float plan.

Equipment and Nomenclature

Label each part of the canoe with the appropriate term (answers on page 12).

Top View

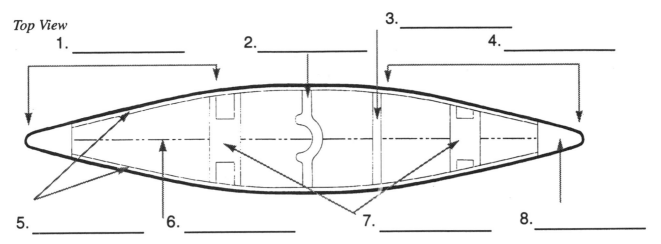

1. _____ 2. _____ 3. _____ 4. _____

5. _____ 6. _____ 7. _____ 8. _____

A. **KEEL LINE.** A real or imaginary line from end to end down the center of the canoe.
B. **GUNWALES (PRONOUNCED GUNNEL)/RAILS.** Reinforcing material along top edges of the sides of the boat.
C. **SEATS.** Used for kneeling support or seating and located at bow and stern for tandem paddlers, center for solo paddlers.
D. **THWARTS.** Gunwale to gunwale (rail to rail) cross braces.
E. **PORTAGE YOKE.** A shoulder rest to aid in canoe portaging.
F. **END DECK.** Triangular reinforcement at the bow and stern.
G. **BOW.** The front or forward part of the boat.
H. **STERN.** The back portion of the boat.

Quick, which direction do paddlers face when paddling the boat above?
Hint: Think about where your feet go if you decide to sit instead of kneel.
With this hint in mind, you'll always be able to decide which end is the bow
and which end is the stern.

Side View

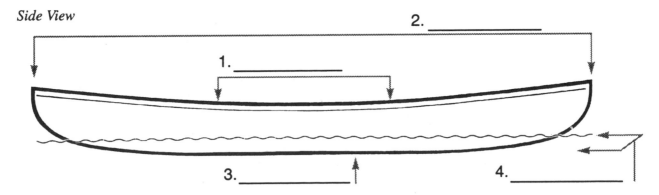

1. _____ 2. _____

3. _____ 4. _____

A. **LENGTH.** Longitudinal measurement from end to end.
B. **DRAFT.** The vertical distance from the bottom of the boat to the waterline.
C. **KEEL LINE.** The longitudinal centerline of the canoe.
D. **AMIDSHIPS.** Midsection of the boat, between the bow and stern.

End View

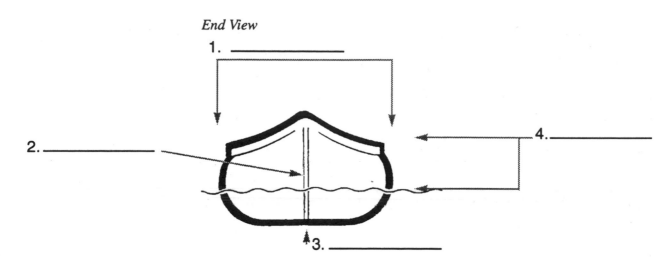

1. _____
2. _____
3. _____
4. _____

A. STEM. Bow or stern vertical edge of the canoe.
B. BEAM. Width of the canoe at amidships.
C. FREEBOARD. The vertical distance from water to the lowest point along the gunwale.
D. KEEL LINE. The longitudinal center line of the canoe.

PADDLE PARTS

Label each part of this bent paddle.

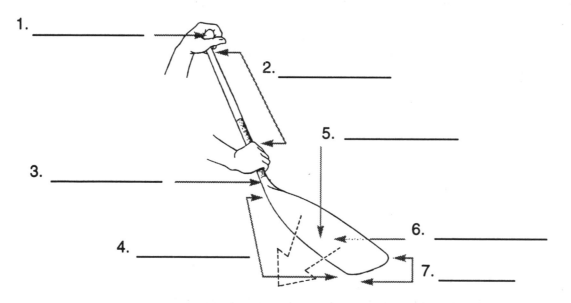

1. _____
2. _____
3. _____
4. _____
5. _____
6. _____
7. _____

A. BLADE. The flat section of the paddle which moves through the water.
B TIP. The blade's bottom edge
C. GRIP. The control handle shaped to fit the paddler's top hand.
D. SHAFT. The section of paddle between the blade and grip.
E. THROAT. The junction between blade and shaft.
F. POWERFACE. The side of the blade catching the water during a forward stroke.
G. BACKFACE. The other side of the blade.

Length is an important canoe measurement; it determines maximum speed and is an indicator of capacity. Longer canoes are faster than shorter ones, but the increased drag of the longer surface area requires more energy to achieve a given speed.

Width and *fullness* give an indication of forward efficiency, seaworthiness, and ability to travel straight or "track." *Narrow*, fine lined, canoes are efficient, requiring less effort at given speeds than wider canoes. They track well, but are not as stable as wider models.

Cross sectional shaping effects stability. *Flat-bottomed* hulls have good initial stability but roll badly in waves. *Rounder bottoms* are less stable when entered, but more stable in heavy seas and generally track well. *Flared hulls* maximize seaworthiness by deflecting waves outward, but make vertical paddle strokes difficult for smaller paddlers. *Tumblehome*, or the inward curvature to the gunwale, increases paddling efficiency by narrowing the boat at the gunwales, making vertical paddle placement easier.

TUMBLEHOME   FLARE

Rocker is the upturn of the stems along the keel line. It affects maneuverability and handling. More rocker allows a canoe to be turned easily. Less stern rocker increases tracking ability but reduces turning ability.

CANOE ROCKER

Select a canoe with volume appropriate to the weight to be carried. Remember that smaller canoes are more efficient at moderate speeds. Lake canoes tend to be long and lean with reduced rocker to combine efficiency and tracking. River canoes need fuller lines and more rocker.

Canoes are made from many materials including aluminum, wood, wood and fabric, fiberglass, sandwiched plastic, and plastic and fabric composites. The material used in construction may be selected based on individual preferences regarding tradition, ruggedness, lightness, performance, and cost.

SELECTING AND SIZING A PADDLE

The paddle transfers our effort into canoe movement. Proper size and selection increases the boat's responsiveness and canoeing fun. Most good paddles have blades about 8 inches wide and 18 to 24 inches long. Shaft length varies according to paddler's torso length and position in canoe.

STRAIGHT AND BENT PADDLES

Canoe paddles are either straight or bent. Straight paddles are more common. The straight design works best for kneeling paddlers, and either blade face may be used.

Sitting paddlers often prefer bent paddles. Bent paddle blades are angled at 10 to 15 degrees to the shaft and may only be used with the bend angled forward (the "V's" open top facing forward). This maximizes forward paddling efficiency but complicates turning strokes and course directions.

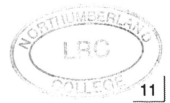

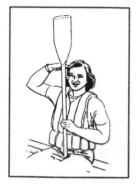

To select the correct length of a canoe paddle, sit upright on a flat surface. Place the paddle grip between your legs and extend the blade upward. The throat of a straight paddle should reach the top of your head. The bent paddle's throat should reach the bridge of your nose. Seating options, canoe type, and load may reduce or increase this optimal length by an inch or two. Once in the canoe, your control (top) hand should be approximately at eye-level with the blade immersed and the paddle vertical.

REVIEW: PADDLES AND CANOES

1. How do you measure for proper paddle length?

2. How do you choose between straight and bent-shaft paddles?

3. Longer canoes have the potential for greater _____ than shorter ones.

4. Describe how a lake canoe should be shaped.

5. Describe how a river canoe should be shaped.

6. Describe the performance differences between canoes with round versus flat bottoms.

7. Describe the performance and paddling differences between canoes with flare versus tumblehome shapes.

Answers to canoe and paddle parts quiz on pages 9 and 10.
Canoe Top View: 1. G; 2. E; 3. D; 4. H; 5. B; 6. A; 7. C; 8. F.
Canoe Side View: 1. D; 2. A; 3. C; 4. B.
Canoe End View: 1. B; 2. A; 3. D; 4. C.
Paddle Parts: 1. C; 2. D; 3. E; 4. A; 5. F; 6. G; 7. B.

Transporting, Carrying, Launching and Boarding

TIE DOWN FOR TRANSPORTATION

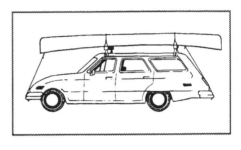

Canoes should be secured amidships to cartop carriers (racks) and both bow and stern tied to the vehicle's bumpers. Use two cross ropes or straps for the racks and canoe ends; secure ropes to bumpers or another solid part of your vehicle to form a "V" (bumper to bow/stern to bumper). Make sure the racks are secure and both the vehicle and racks are sturdy enough for the load.

It is recommended that you use straps made of high strength nylon webbing and strong buckles. If ropes are used, use proper knots such as the "truckers hitch," "half hitches," and "bowline." (See the ACA publication *Knots for Paddlers*.) Avoid the use of bungee or elastic cords. They may allow the boat to shift and fall off the car at highway speeds.

LIFTING THE CANOE AND THE OVERHEAD CARRY

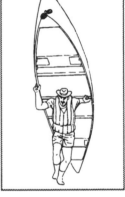

With the canoe on the ground, bend at the knees and grasp the near gunwale on either side of the center. Lift the canoe with both legs until the bottom rests on both thighs. Reach to the far gunwale/rail with one hand. With a backwards, rocking motion, bounce the canoe upwards while pulling it over the head, comfortably adjusting the hands. Rest the portage yoke or center seat on the back of the neck and across the shoulders. If the canoe is too heavy to lift, the load can be reduced by leaving one end on the ground while you roll the other end overhead.

ONE SHOULDER CARRY

Lightweight solo canoes can be carried short distances, stern forward, with the center point of one gunwale resting on a shoulder, the supporting arm grasping the center seat for control. The lift is similar to lifting the canoe onto one's shoulders, but the canoe isn't rolled as far.

TWO-PERSON CARRY

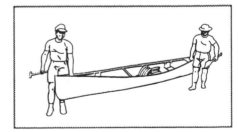

With a person on opposite sides, canoes can be carried upright by grasping under the boat's end, or by holding the grab handles or end deck.

Launch the canoe by placing one end into the water and "feeding" the boat hand over hand until it is floating fully. Do not let go of the boat!

BOARDING

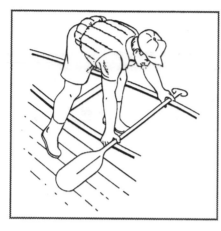

Launch the canoe and bring it parallel to the shore in deep enough water so the canoe will float when loaded. When on moving water, the upstream end needs to be held tight to shore, keeping the canoe from spinning into the current. In shallows the canoe is walked from shore into ankle deep water. Cargo is always loaded before paddlers. Trim the canoe level by equal load distribution.

To enter the canoe, lay the paddle across the gunwales with the blade to shore. Facing forward, grasp both gunwales and lean the canoe to shore until the paddle blade braces against the shore or bottom. Transfer your weight slowly onto the bottom center of the canoe placing one foot at a time. Maintain three points of contact when boarding and moving about in a canoe. Either two hands and one foot, or both feet and one hand should be in contact with the craft at all times. Board the canoe directly into your paddling position whenever possible.

For maximum stability, kneel. Kneeling is sitting with the knees down, spread as far apart as is comfortable; this stance increases stability and paddling power. Lean back against the seat or thwart. The toes may be pointed toward the stern (aft) or placed against the bottom to elevate the ankles. Comfort suggests alternating toe positions and using knee pads.

When paddling tandem, the stern paddler generally enters the canoe first. The stern's stance is generally wider and more stable, and the stern can easily view the bow paddler's entry.

SITTING

Some canoes are designed with low mounted bucket seats for sitting paddlers. While the paddler's stability and reach is reduced, the sitting position is more comfortable for long paddling sessions, and often selected for lake travel. Foot braces improve stability and paddling efficiency.

The Strokes

Paddling is the art and science of moving a canoe through the water. The key is to maximize body and paddle efficiency in order to move your boat. For best effect, keep the paddle blade at right angles to the direction of travel; efficiency fades quickly as the angle changes. Keep the shaft vertical to the water surface when moving forward or in reverse. Keep the shaft horizontal on sweep strokes which are used to turn the boat. Focus on moving the boat toward your paddle.

HOLDING THE PADDLE

Space the grip hand and shaft hand shoulder width apart when holding a paddle. Arms should remain virtually straight. This allows the blade to be kept vertical longer for more efficient paddling and encourages using the larger torso muscles in your back to power the canoe. Bent arms use smaller, less efficient muscles.

PADDLE STROKE NOMENCLATURE

Paddle strokes have three phases: catch, propulsion, and recovery. The paddle enters the water during the catch at right angles to the direction of travel or resistance. During the propulsion phase the canoe moves in a given direction. Recovery may be made in or out of the water. The paddle is usually feathered, with the blade edge leading, during the recovery phase.

STROKE TERMINOLOGY

To help simultaneously explain strokes for left handed and right handed paddlers, generic terms are used to describe the paddle, boat, and hands. "Onside" refers to the side of the canoe where the solo paddler's hands are found during a forward stroke. The opposite side of the canoe is termed the "offside." For tandem canoes, onside and offside are determined by the bow paddler's hand position.

   The hand on the grip of the paddle which controls blade angle is called the "control hand." The thumb on the control hand is the "control thumb." The hand on the shaft of the paddle which serves as a lever is called the "shaft hand" and the arm is the "shaft arm."

THE STROKES

Description of the basic strokes follow. When the strokes are actually used, they may be modified or combined to achieve the movement or reaction desired of the canoe. It is helpful to have a canoe paddle in one's hands as the description of the strokes are read. All strokes can be practiced while sitting in a straight-backed chair.

   The following illustrations show solo paddlers, but all of the strokes can be adopted for tandem canoeing. Tandem paddlers work together as a team. The bow paddler sets the cadence, the stern reads and follows the bow's lead. The bow, however, should feel the rhythm of the boat and listen for instructions from the stern. Bow and stern paddle on opposite sides of the canoe. If the bow switches paddling sides, the stern does, too. Paddling on opposite sides in cadence eliminates unwanted sideways "fishtailing" and increases stability and forward efficiency. Ideally, tandem partners should both kneel or both sit, and use similar paddles. Remember, it takes time and communication to build a tandem team.

Because canoes tend to turn, we first present strokes which *cause* them to spin. These include the draw, pushaway, pry, cross draw, sweep, and reverse sweep. Learning these strokes will give you control of your craft. Forward and correction strokes are presented last.

DRAW

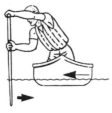

The draw moves the canoe abeam (sideways) towards the paddle, or can turn the canoe when used at either end. The draw begins as the paddler turns onside, lining shoulders with the centerline of the boat. The catch begins off the paddler's hip, with both arms extended and the control thumb pointed aft. The blade is parallel to the keel line, the powerface toward the canoe.

The draw is powered by pulling the onside hip towards the paddle, keeping the control arm stiff and bending the shaft arm slightly. As the canoe approaches the blade, the power phase of the draw stroke ends. To recover, rotate the control thumb away from you, slicing the edge of the blade through the water to the catch position. Point the control thumb aft to begin the next draw. This is an "in-water recovery."

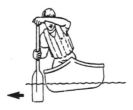

Keep the paddle vertical in the water to increase efficiency. A series of short, quick draw strokes is preferred. Hint: Moving the boat to the paddle creates the illusion of trying to push water under the canoe. Think of your paddle as a broom and you are sweeping dirt under a carpet!

PUSHAWAY

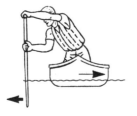

The pushaway is the opposite of the draw, moving the canoe abeam (sideways) away from the paddle.

The catch is at the paddler's hip, alongside the canoe, with the control thumb pointed aft, the blade parallel to the keel. With both arms slightly bent, push the blade's backface away from the canoe using torso action and by straightening both arms.

Recover to successive pushaways with an in-water recovery. Begin by turning the control thumb outwards and slicing the paddle back to the catch position, where the thumb is turned aft again. Keep the strokes short and the paddle shaft vertical.

The pry forcefully moves the canoe abeam (sideways) away from the paddling side.

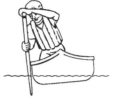

The catch is alongside the canoe with the blade parallel to the keel and the shaft angled under the canoe slightly. The paddler rotates to the paddle side, both arms slightly bent with the control hand extended across the gunwale, thumb pointing aft. Turning the torso forward forces the control hand inwards, levering the blade's backface out and "prying" the canoe away from the blade.

Keep the pry short with the shaft nearly vertical through out. Use an in-water recovery between strokes. Turn the control thumb outwards and slice the paddle back to the catch position.

The cross draw moves the canoe to the bow paddler's offside. It is used as a turning stroke in solo canoes, and by the bow paddler in tandem canoes .

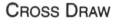

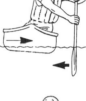

The cross draw is executed without the paddler changing hand positions on the paddle, yet is performed on the opposite side of the canoe. The paddler rotates sharply away from the onside with the shaft arm extended forward. The blade is carried across the bow and placed abeam and away from the paddler's offside knee, powerface pointing to offside gunwale. Paddle shaft is vertical at the catch, shaft arm is straight, and control arm is bent with the control thumb pointed forward and away from the bow. Using good torso rotation, turn the boat toward the blade by pulling the paddle to the bow of the canoe.

The sweep turns the bow away from the paddle while maintaining forward momentum. The reverse sweep turns the bow toward the paddle and slows forward momentum. This is true for solo, bow and stern paddlers, but in tandem boats, one paddler executes the sweep and the other a reverse sweep (descriptions follow) to spin the boat.

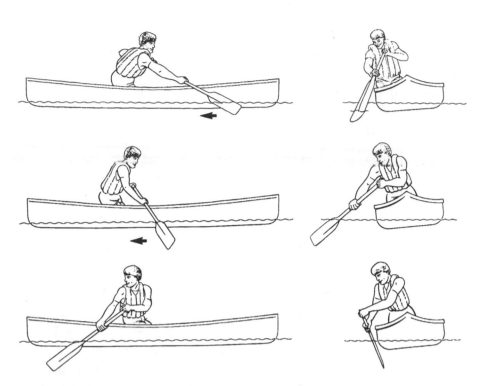

The paddle shaft is held horizontally with the shaft arm straight and the control arm bent. The control hand is held low with the thumb pointing up. The paddler leans forward slightly, rotating the torso 45 degrees to the offside (the shaft arm's shoulder reaches forward). At the catch, the paddle blade (not the shaft) is vertical in the water alongside the bow. With both arms rigid and using torso rotation to power the stroke, the blade arcs in a semi-circle to the stern. Watch the paddle blade as it moves through the semi-circle to help generate torso motion. Both hands should extend across the gunwale, the shaft arm bending slightly only as the blade nears the stern. Bending the arm at this point is important to protect the shoulder from potential injury.

The "horizontal recovery" returns the paddle from stroke's end to the catch position. At the end of the forward sweep, rotate the control thumb forward and slice the blade forward with locked elbows while using torso rotation to turn the body and get ready for the next stroke. The blade should be flat above the water with the powerface up. When the blade has been carried to the catch position, rotate the control thumb up to orient the blade for another sweep.

THE SOLO REVERSE SWEEP

The reverse sweep turns the canoe sharply onside, reducing forward momentum.

The solo paddler's body rotates onside with the onside shoulder turned towards the stern. The paddle shaft is held horizontally with the control arm bent, the control thumb pointing up. The shaft arm is slightly bent with the shaft hand well behind the paddler's hip. The blade is placed vertically near the aft side of the canoe. The shaft arm extends aft, and, after the start, locks into an almost straight position throughout the stroke. With the paddler con-

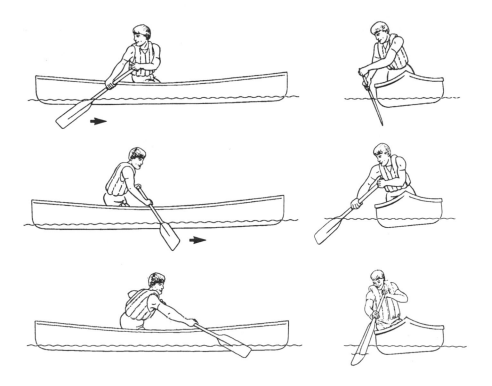

centrating looking at the blade, the torso uncoils, arcing the blade forward, and pushing on the blade's backface against the water. The bow swings onside with the stern swinging away.

A horizontal recovery is used between reverse sweeps. At the end of the reverse sweep, turn your control thumb forward to feather the paddle. Slice the blade backwards with locked elbows, using torso rotation to turn the body. The blade should be flat above the water with the powerface up. When the blade reaches the catch position, turn the control thumb up to orient the blade for another reverse sweep.

SOLO SWEEPS VERSUS BOW AND TANDEM SWEEPS

The solo paddler's sweep arcs 180 degrees and travels from "tip to tip," or end to end, of the canoe. Tandem paddlers sweep 90 degrees and work only in the area from their hips to the tip of the boat that is closest to them. Tandem sweeps are termed "bow" or "stern sweeps," or "bow" or "stern reverse sweeps."

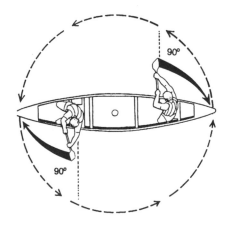

To turn to the onside, stern paddlers sweep from abeam the paddler's hip to the stern of the canoe, or from "hip to tip." Bow paddlers sweep "tip to hip," beginning the sweep at the bow. To spin to the offside, reverse the direction of the sweeps, making sure to remain in the tip to hip area.

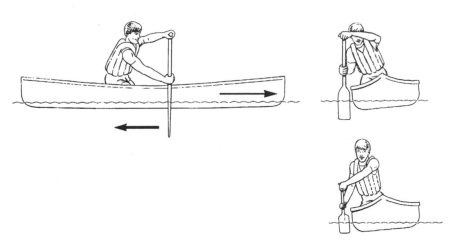

The forward stroke moves the canoe forward and is the key to successful canoeing. It must be parallel to the keel line, as close to the keel as possible, and relatively short to keep the blade vertical through the power phase.

The paddler rotates the torso 45 degrees offside, extending both arms forward and both hands across the gunwale. Position the shaft arm outside the gunwale with the shaft vertical. The control hand is positioned on the grip with the thumb pointed out and must be "stacked" above the shaft hand to keep the paddle vertical. The catch should be about two feet forward of the onside knee.

The power phase of the forward stroke is driven by torso rotation. Uncoil the torso from the 45-degree catch position to face forward. Keep both arms straight. The stroke should be parallel to the keel line, *not* to the gunwale.

When kneeling, the power phase ends when the shaft reaches the knee. Carrying the stroke farther back wastes energy by lifting water and turning the canoe. Use the horizontal recovery or in-water recovery to reposition for additional strokes.Paddling when sitting limits torso rotation. With the catch just forward of the paddler's knee when seated, the power phase extends from knee to hips. For bent paddles the horizontal recovery is preferable to the in-water recovery.

BACK STROKE

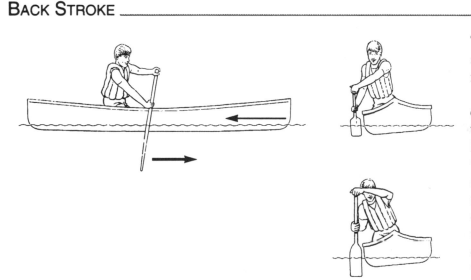

The back stroke is used to stop forward motion or to move the canoe backwards.

The paddler rotates 45 degrees onside and places the paddle just behind the hip with the paddle shaft vertical. Both arms are slightly bent. Both hands are across the gunwale with the control hand out slightly farther than the shaft hand. The control thumb points outwards.

Using torso rotation, drive the backface forward towards the bow until the blade is even with the paddler's knee. For an in-water recovery, rotate the control thumb aft to slice back to the catch position.

"J" STROKE

The "J" stroke, a modification of the forward stroke, is used by solo and stern paddlers to keep the canoe going straight. At the conclusion of a forward stroke with the blade fully in the water, rotate the control thumb outwards and down. The shaft hand pushes the blades away from the boat. The amount of "J" required to keep the canoe on a straight course may vary 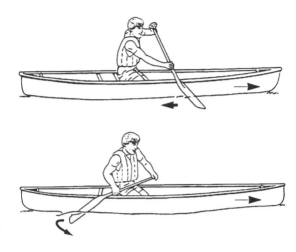 from stroke to stroke, but should generally be quite slight. This stroke may be a challenging stroke to master.

STERN PRY AND STERN DRAW

These pry and draw strokes are used as corrective steering or rudder strokes for a boat underway. At the conclusion of a forward stroke, with the blade fully in the water, rotate the control thumb up. Position the paddle shaft along the side of the canoe for a stern pry or away from the canoe for a stern draw.

MANEUVERS

SPINS

Spins rotate the canoe on its center. Solo canoes spin with sweeps or reverse sweeps. Tandem canoes spin with several mixtures of bow and stern strokes. A few combinations are:
- A bow reverse sweep and stern sweep.
- A bow sweep and stern reverse sweep.
- A bow draw in unison with a stern draw.
- A bow pushaway or pry in unison with a stern pushaway or pry.
- A bow cross draw in unison with a stern pry or pushaway.

TURNS UNDERWAY

To turn the canoe while moving, select strokes which reduce drag. While a variety of strokes may turn the canoe, the following combinations are most effective at maintaining forward momentum:
- Turn solo canoes to the onside using a draw stroke to the bow.
- Turn solo canoes to the offside using a sweep.
- Turn tandem canoes to the onside by combining a bow draw with a stern sweep.
- Turn tandem canoes to the offside using a bow sweep with a stern "J."

Abeams move the canoe sideways without turning it. Abeams are useful for leaving and approaching shore and avoiding obstacles in moving water. Draws, pushaways, prys, and cross draws move the solo canoe abeam. Tandem paddlers may use a variety of combinations including:

■ A bow draw with a stern pry or pushaway to move the canoe to the onside.
■ A bow pushaway or cross draw with a stern draw for an offside move.

DIFFERENT STROKES FOR TANDEM FOLKS

Name the stroke. Also note the direction the canoe will travel. The arrows represent the directions of the paddles.

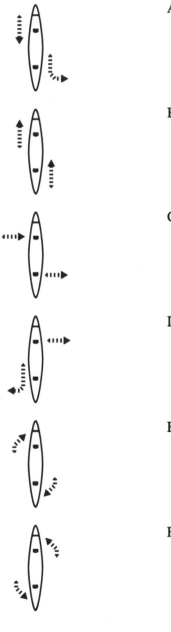

A. Bow

Stern

Direction

B. Bow

Stern

Direction

C. Bow

Stern

Direction

D. Bow

Stern

Direction

E. Bow

Stern

Direction

F. Bow

Stern

Direction

Canoeing on Moving Water

Strokes and maneuvers executed and developed on flatwater provide an excellent foundation for paddling on moving water. In addition to basic strokes, you need to understand river dynamics and how to read the river. You also should understand the force of moving water. A gallon of water weighs about 8 pounds. The faster water flows, the greater kinetic energy, or force, it creates. Hundreds, even thousands, of pounds of force can be created against a pinned or trapped person or boat.

Understanding the characteristics of the moving water environment allows you to develop understanding and respect. Take a river paddling course and learn about moving water before venturing out.

HOW TO READ A RIVER

DOWNSTREAM "V'S."   Surface feature of the river formed by two parallel obstructions, indicating a clear, deep water path. Water lines formed off the obstructions join downstream, thus pointing the way.

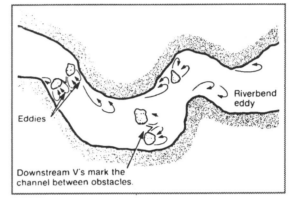

Downstream V's mark the channel between obstacles.

STANDING WAVES.   Formed usually at the base of a drop or downstream "V" caused by accelerating water coming in contact with slower moving water downstream. Standing waves are a series of waves that are stationary, but the water is moving. Big waves are sometimes referred to as "haystacks."

EDDY.   An obstruction above the water's surface forces moving water to go around it. As the downstream flow of water fills in behind the obstruction it creates an upstream, relatively slow movement of the water called an eddy. Eddies provide stopping spots for paddlers to rest and look downstream.

EDDY LINE.   The border between the eddy current and main current flow distinguishing a change of current direction.

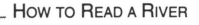

PILLOW.   A smooth, shallow mound of moving water covering a structure just below the surface. The mound of water is not sufficiently deep to paddle over. A white wave or depression just downstream is a clue of trouble upstream. Remember in river paddling, "pillows are stuffed with rocks."

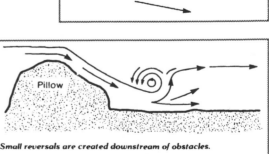

Small reversals are created downstream of obstacles.

HOLE.   A depression in the river's surface caused by water flowing over a rock or ledge.

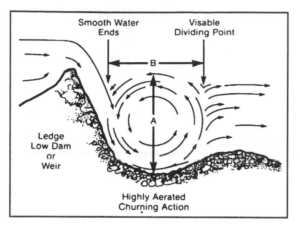

Smooth Water Ends

Visable Dividing Point

B

A

Ledge Low Dam or Weir

Highly Aerated Churning Action

HYDRAULIC. Water flowing over an obstacle and landing on surface water below creates a depression. Downstream surface water rushes upstream to fill in this depression creating a vertical whirlpool effect. When the hydraulic is large enough to trap and recirculate a boat, it is referred to as a "keeper."

LOW HEAD DAM. A man made river hazard. Difficult to detect from upstream. It can be recognized by a horizontal line across the river called a "horizon line." These structures can create keeper hydraulics which are difficult to escape. Low head dams are often called "Drowning Machines." All dams should be portaged.

HYPOTHERMIA. See page 6 for more on protecting yourself from the cold.

HIGH WATER. Moving water has awesome power, especially in high water. Learn river reading and moving water maneuvers before you go out.

STRAINERS. Obstacles in the river such as trees, cables, fences, brush, drainage grates, or anything that can trap debris while allowing water to pass through. The force of moving water can pin people and canoes against strainers leading to serious injury and even death. Avoid strainers at all costs! Do not underestimate their danger.

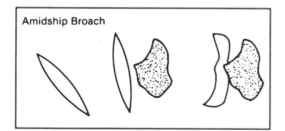

Amidship Broach

BROACHING. A broach occurs when the current pushes a boat sideways against an immovable object causing the boat to stall or stop. To guard against broaching, lean the boat toward the object. Leaning toward the rock or obstruction allows upstream water to flow under the boat "lifting" it around the obstruction and potential danger.

MOVING WATER MANEUVERS

Paddlers use specific maneuvers to get around on moving water. Because of the remarkable forces created by moving water, paddler strength is no match. Instead, learn to harness the power of the river. Learn to finesse the river with cool, efficient, and fun river maneuvers like the ones listed below.

EDDY TURN

Boat speed, boat angle, and boat lean (heeling) are key components to entering an eddy. Enter the eddy with enough speed to cross the eddy line, but not so much that you fly out the other side. Approach the eddy so you will enter it at about a 45 degree angle. Heel the canoe just like leaning a bicycle through a turn. Boat lean will stop your boat from capsizing to the outside of the turn as the boat enters the slower moving, upstream flowing eddy.

A peelout is fast, exciting, and sometimes the only way to exit an eddy. Just like the eddy turn coming in, boat speed, boat angle, and boat lean are key components to the peelout. Exit the eddy with enough speed to cross the eddy line. Go too slow, and you may not be able to cross the eddy line. Cross the eddy line at a 45- to 90-degree angle, depending on the speed of the mainstream current; the

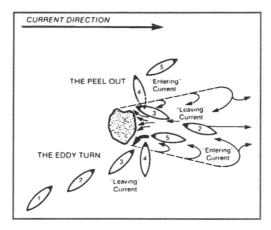

faster the current, the closer to 45 degrees you should be. Lean the canoe just like leaning a bicycle through a turn. Boat lean resists capsizing upstream as the boat enters the faster downstream moving current.

Ferrying is a method of crossing current without getting swept downstream. The ferry uses the water's energy deflected off the side of the canoe. This force, balanced against upstream paddling, results in movement of the boat across the current. Ferrying is helpful to line up for running downstream "V's", or for maneuvering around hazards like rocks and strainers.

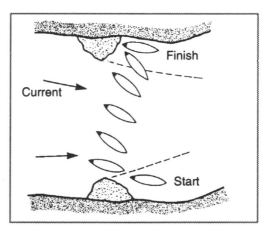

The key to successful ferrying is in both boat angle and speed. The slower the current the greater the angle. To ferry, point the upstream end of the canoe slightly towards the shore you wish to reach and, holding that angle, paddle upstream into the current. Continue paddling until you reach the other side.

There are upstream and downstream ferries. Typically, the easiest ferry is the upstream, or forward, ferry. The bow of the canoe is pointed upstream and the paddlers primarily use forward strokes. This makes it easier to see the current and make adjustments for a successful ferry. The bow paddler provides power while the stern paddler is chiefly responsible for angle and direction.

For the downstream or back ferry, the bow of the canoe points downstream and the paddlers primarily use back strokes. This allows the paddlers to see better where the canoe is going or what it is avoiding. The stern paddler provides power while the bow paddler is chiefly responsible for angle and direction. This is typically a more difficult maneuver to execute.

Answers to page 22: **A.** Forward / J-stroke / Forward. **B.** Reverse / Reverse / Backward or Stopping. **C.** Draw / Pry or Pushaway / Onside Abeam. **D.** Pry or Pushaway / J-stroke / Offside turn underway. **E.** Reverse Sweep / Sweep / Onside spin (Counterclockwise). **F.** Reverse Sweep / Sweep / Onside spin (Clockwise)

Know your put-in and your take-out before you begin. Travel in at least groups of three boats. Keep the boat behind you in sight. The lead boat should be able to recognize and avoid hazards: low-head dams, high rapids, and hydraulics.

Upstream V's indicate rocks.

The river is usually faster on the outside of a bend. When you approach obstructions, set your course in advance using good ferry angles. When in doubt, scout from the shore and walk around (portage).

Trees and other objects in the river are potential strainers. Steer clear of them.

LOOK OUT!
If the river disappears, you may be approaching a steep drop or waterfall. Scout and portage. Run only if properly trained and equipped using all precautions.

If capsized, stay on the upstream side of the canoe. Keep your feet up. Never stand in moving water unless it is less than knee deep. Set a rescue point with a knowledgeable paddler on shore before running any difficult drop. If you are not prepared to swim the rapid, don't paddle it!

Broken arrows: Portage.
Solid arrows: Preferred course.
Dotted arrow: Optional course.

Canoeing on Lakes and State Waterways

Many lakes and rivers are marked with information and regulatory signs and buoys indicating restricted or hazardous areas. It's important to keep in mind that not all hazards are marked. The good flat-water paddler always obeys these signs:

 CONTROLLED AREA. Look in the circle for further information. These are found at speed zones, no fishing areas, no anchoring areas, ski zones, no wake zones, etc.

 BOATS KEEP OUT. The nature of the danger may be placed around the outside of the crossed diamond. These may mark waterfalls, dams, swim areas, or rapids.

 DANGER—USE CAUTION. This may mark construction areas, reefs, shoals, or sunken objects.

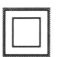 **INFORMATION.** These tell directions, distances, and other non-regulatory messages.

PADDLING REVIEW QUESTIONS

1. What is the proper hand positioning on the paddle?

2. Why are feathered recoveries important?

3. Name 3 key points about tandem paddling.

4. With the bow paddling on right, the stern on left, list combinations turning the canoe offside (counterclockwise).

5. As above, list onside (clockwise) combinations.

6. What is the purpose of the "J" stroke?

7. Why do we try to keep the paddle shaft vertical on draws, pushaways, forward, and back strokes?

8. Why do we hold the shaft nearly horizontal for sweeps and reverse sweeps?

9. What phase of the paddle stroke transfers the most force to the water?

10. What are three common factors in eddy turns and peelouts?

11. What force aids in ferrying a boat?

Safety and Rescue

RESCUE

Capsizing is part of the sport of canoeing. Boaters should be able to handle their own craft in capsizes and swamps and aid others in need. Always be prepared to swim. Dress properly and wear your life jacket. Being prepared is the first step to rescue. Self rescue is the quickest and surest method.

SELF RESCUE

The simplest form of self rescue is wading or swimming to the closest safe shore with the canoe. In moving water, stay on the upstream side of the boat; this prevents entrapment of your body between the canoe and downstream obstructions. On a lake, if the self-rescue involves a long distance to shore, you may want to re-enter the canoe even if it is partially filled with water. Whenever possible, stay with the canoe. It provides positive flotation, and a large object is more visible to rescuers as well as power boats that might otherwise run you down accidentally.

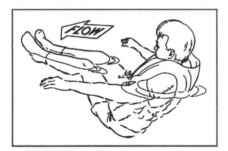

In some moving water mishaps, it may be advisable to release the canoe and swim to shore. The safest method of swimming in moving water is on your back with your feet downstream. Keep your head up and your toes at the water's surface. Use your feet to fend off rocks. Position your body to ferry into the nearest eddy using strong kicks and your arms to help direct your movement. Do not stand up in the current until you are in water less than knee deep. Standing in fast moving, water that is more than knee deep may result in injury or drowning due to a foot entrapment.

EMPTYING THE CANOE

To empty a capsized boat that is floating upside down in water where you can stand, raise one end of the canoe to the water's surface. Push down on the opposite end of the boat while lifting one gunwale to break the water's suction. With the canoe still upside down, raise the canoe out of the water with help from a partner on the opposite end. After allowing several seconds for the canoe to drain, roll the canoe to the upright position on the surface of the water. In deeper water, a canoe over canoe rescue is most effective. See below.

RE-ENTERING THE CANOE IN DEEP WATER

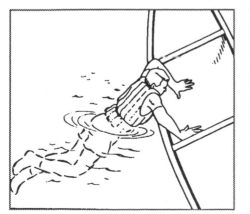

If shore access is not possible, you can re-enter the canoe from deep water. Begin by placing your hands on both gunwales near the wide section of the canoe, although hand placement may vary due to canoe width and stability, arm length, and paddler strength. There should be space available for your body in the section to be entered. Pressing down with both hands and using a strong kick, lift the body upwards until the hips are across the nearest gunwale. Roll onto your back and sit on the bottom of the canoe before bringing your legs in. Hand paddle the canoe if necessary to retrieve paddles and gear. Swamped canoes may be paddled to shore with paddles, or if necessary with your hands. They may also be bailed.

A second canoe can assist by holding the gunwale opposite the side being re-entered, thereby stabilizing the boat. Tandem paddlers help stabilize the boat for their partners and re-enter one at a time from opposite sides.

RESCUING OTHERS

When in position to assist others, use this RESCUE SEQUENCE: Reach, Throw, Row, Go.

REACH. Often reaching a hand to a swimming paddler can bring them safely to shore or to your canoe's gunwale. A paddle can extend your reach safely.

THROW. When the swimmer is too far away to reach with a paddle or pole, a thrown float or rope can often aid the paddler's rescue.

ROW. If the swimmer is beyond range to be thrown a rescue device, the rescuer should maneuver his or her boat to assist in position where a reach or throw technique is possible. A rescuer in a boat is safer than a swimming one.

GO. As a last option, a trained and properly equipped rescuer can swim to the aid of the swimmers. Bystanders should call for help.

BOAT BUMP RESCUE

When paddling to rescue a swimmer, tow the swimmer at the stern of your canoe while bumping the swamped boat to calm water at a close shore.

BOAT OVER BOAT RESCUE

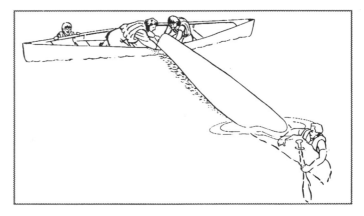

In open water with a second canoe to assist as a rescue boat, a boat over boat rescue is quick and very effective. Assume a tandem boat has capsized:

Capsized paddler #1 holds onto the end of the rescue canoe. Capsized paddler #2 helps line the capsized boat up perpendicular to the rescue boat forming a "T," and remains in the position at the bottom of the "T." The rescuers at the top of the "T" hold onto the capsized boat's end allowing capsized paddler #2 (bottom of the "T") to push down on the boat and break the vacuum. This action raises the end near the rescue boat up and out of the water. With capsizes involving lightweight people, more than one person may be needed to push down on the end of the boat.

Keeping the boat upside down, the rescuers pull the boat up and across their craft until it balances on their gunwales forming an "+". Be careful not to pinch fingers between the two boats. The capsized paddlers should keep hold of the canoe as it is pulled in, and move to a stabilizing position on the rescue boat.

The rescuers allow the boat to drain, then flip it upright position while continuing to balance it across both gunwales.

The rescuers slide the canoe into the water without losing contact. They stabilize the craft, gunwale to gunwale, with their own boat. The capsized paddlers re-enter with either a deep water re-entry or a rescue sling entry.

RESCUE SLING

A method that enables a paddler to climb into a boat with little difficulty is the rescue sling technique. Loop over the gunwale a section of line or webbing long enough to hang into the water. Secure the loop across the boat onto a second boat, or if a second paddler is in the water to help stabilize, secure the loop directly onto a thwart. The paddler then places a foot in the loop using it like a stirrup. Lifting the hips above the gunwale line, the paddler climbs into the center of the boat.

EXPOSURE IN WATER

When paddlers are unable to re-enter their craft quickly, they may risk hypothermia especially if water or air temperature is low. The Heat Escape Lessening Posture (HELP) and HUDDLE position minimize heat loss in cold water.

HELP POSITION

The HELP position protects the highest heat loss areas of the body: the head, neck, underarms, and groin area. This technique is possible only when wearing a life jacket. To adopt the HELP position, the individual swimmer:

- Crosses the legs at the ankles and pulls the legs toward the chest.
- Crosses the arms at the chest being careful to protect the area under the arms, or holds the neck with the hands for additional protection.
- Keeps the head out of the water.

HUDDLE

A group of paddlers huddling together conserve body temperature more efficiently than floating alone. To HUDDLE, body to body contact is critical. Form a circle, placing smaller or weaker individuals inside. Wrap arms around one another with legs together.

RESCUE QUESTIONS

1. Name the steps in the rescue sequence.

2. Why stay with the canoe when capsized or swamped?

3. Why is it hazardous to stand in moving water?

4. Describe two techniques for minimizing heat loss in cold water.

ABEAM. At a right angle to the keel line.

ABOARD. On, in or into a boat.

AFLOAT. On the water.

AFT. A term describing direction toward the rear or stern of a boat.

AGROUND. Touching bottom.

AMIDSHIP. Describing the midsection of a vessel.

ASTERN. Aft or toward the stern.

BACKFACE. The side of the paddle blade opposite the powerface.

BAIL. Removing water from the canoe with sponge, scoop or bailer.

BANG PLATE. A strip of abrasion resistant material added to protect canoe stems.

BEAM. Vessel's width amidship.

BLADE. Wide, flat paddle part transferring force to water, flat section of paddle.

BOIL. A mound of water deflected up by underwater obstructions.

BOW. The forward part of a canoe, front of the boat.

BRACING. A paddle placement resisting capsize.

BROACH. To be turned broadside by wind, wave, or current.

BUOYANCY CHAMBER. Flotation tanks usually at ends of the boat.

CAPSIZE. To turn the canoe over in the water.

CATCH. The part of a paddle stroke placing the blade in water.

CHANNEL. A route through obstructions in a section of river.

CHINE. The transition from hull sidewall to bottom.

CHUTE. A narrow channel between obstructions with fast water.

CONTROL HAND. The hand on the paddle grip.

CONTROL THUMB. The control hand thumb; keys paddle orientation.

DECK. A permanent hull or compartment cover.

DEPTH. The vertical distance from canoe gunwales to center line.

DIFFICULTY RATING. The rating of a river section's navigability.

DOWNSTREAM "V." Formed when there are two obstructions and water passes between both to form a "v" which points downstream.

DRAFT. The depth of water a canoe draws.

DROP. A steep sudden slope in a river.

EDDY. The area behind an obstruction in current with still or upstream water flow.

EDDY LINE. The line which separates the eddy from the main current.

EDDY TURN. Utilizing current flow to turn into an eddy.

END DECK. A triangular plate joining gunwales at the canoe end.

END LINE. Rope connected to each end of the canoe; also called painters.

FALLS. Drops where water falls free.

FEATHER. To move the paddle by leading with one edge, thus reducing the drag caused by air or wind during the recovery phase.

FERRY. Maneuver in which a paddler uses the force of the water to move the canoe sideways across the current.

FLARE. Outward broadening canoe cross sectional shape.

FLATWATER. Lake or river water without rapids.

FREEBOARD. The vertical distance from gunwale to waterline.

GRIP. The top of the paddle shaft shaped for the control hand.

GUNWALE OR GUNNEL. The top edge of canoe sides, also called rails.

HAYSTACK. Standing waves below a chute where water flow slows.

HEEL. Tipping the canoe sideways purposefully or by wave action.

HULL. The body of a watercraft.

HYDRAULIC. Turbulence caused by water flowing over an obstacle.

HYPOTHERMIA. Physical condition that occurs when the body loses heat faster than it can produce it.

KEEL. The longitudinal centerline of a canoe.

KEEPER. A hydraulic that holds objects in recirculating water.

LEDGE. A projecting rock layer partially damming water flow.

LINING. Working canoes up or downstream with lines from shore.

LOW HEAD DAM. A fixed obstruction across a stream or river in which water drops over the crest creating a hydraulic that can trap and recirculate objects.

OFFSIDE. The canoe side opposite the solo or bow paddler's shaft hand on a forward stroke.

ONSIDE. The solo or bow paddler's paddle side for a normal forward stroke.

PAINTER. A line attached to canoe's bow or stern, also called an END LINE.

PEELOUT. Turning downstream from an eddy.

PFD. A Personal Flotation Device. A life jacket.

PILLOW. A boil where water deflects upwards from an obstruction.

PORTAGE. Carrying the canoe around or over obstructions.

PORTAGE YOKE. A shoulder rest aiding canoe portaging.

POWERFACE. The face of the blade that pushes against the water on a forward stroke.

RAILS. Same as gunwales, reinforcing at canoe top edge.

RAPIDS. River section with steep fast flow around obstructions.

RECOVERY. Moving the paddle from stroke end to the next catch.

RIFFLES. Water flow across shallows causing small waves.

RIVER LEFT. The left side of the river as you face downstream.

RIVER RIGHT. The right side of the river as you face downstream.

ROCKER. The upward curve of a canoe's keel line at either or both ends.

RUDDER. A stern pry or draw to control direction.

SHAFT. Slender tubular portion of the paddle connecting blade and grip.

SLACK WATER. River flow without riffle or rapids.

SLALOM. White water course requiring maneuver through gates.

SLICE. Edgewise movement of the paddle blade through water.

STANDING WAVE. A wave occurring where current decelerates; also called a hay stack.

STEM. Either vertical end of a canoe.

STERN. The rear portion of a boat.

STOPPER. A hydraulic that arrests forward momentum.

STOW. Secure gear in a boat.

STRAINER. A obstruction in moving water which allows water to pass through but stops and holds objects such as boats and people.

SWAMP. To sink by filling with water.

SWEEP BOAT. The assigned last canoe in a group of paddlers.

TIP. The bottom edge of the paddle blade.

THROAT. The transitional area where paddle blade and shaft meet.

THWART. A structural brace running gunwale to gunwale in open canoes.

TRIM. Balancing a boat so it sits level on water.

TRIP LEADER. An experienced and qualified paddler leading the group on an outing.

TROUGH. The depression between waves.

TUMBLEHOME. Inward curvature of canoe sides at the gunwales.

UPSTREAM "V." Formed by an obstruction in the water which creates a "V" that points upstream.

WATERLINE. The intersection of hull and water surface.

WHITEWATER. Aerated rapids.

Bibliography

Foster, Tom & Kel Kelly. *Catch Every Eddy, Surf Every Wave.* Outdoor Centre of New England.

Glaros, Lou and Charlie Wilson. *FreeStyle Paddling.* Menasha Ridge Press.

Gullion, Laurie. *ACA Canoeing and Kayaking Instructor's Manual.* Menasha Ridge Press.

Gullion, Laurie. *Canoeing.* Human Kinetics Press.

Walbridge, Charlie. *ACA Knots for Paddlers.* Menasha Ridge Press.

Resource Organizations

AMERICAN CANOE ASSOCIATION, 7432 Alban Station, Suite B-226, Springfield, VA 22150, (703) 452-0141.

AMERICAN WHITEWATER AFFILIATION, Box 79, Phoenicia, NY 23445.

NATIONAL ASSOCIATION OF STATE BOATING LAW ADMINISTRATORS, P. O. Box 8510, Lexington, KY 40533, (606) 244-8242.

PROFESSIONAL PADDLESPORTS ASSOCIATION, P. O. Box 248, Butler, KY 41006, (606) 472-2205.